Step Approach: A Guide And Instructions To Walking Benefits And Healthy Living

Edan Allen

Table of Content

Introduction

Embarking on a journey through the world of walking steps unveils a fascinating exploration of movement, rhythm, and mindfulness. From the simplicity of placing one foot in front of the other to the intricate techniques of various walking disciplines, each step offers a gateway to physical health, mental clarity, and spiritual connection. Join me as we delve into the art and science of walking steps, uncovering the myriad benefits and techniques that enrich our daily strides.

Walking steps encompass a rich tapestry of practices, ranging from the basic act of walking for transportation to specialized disciplines like mindful walking, power walking, and walking meditation. Each approach offers unique benefits and insights into the human experience.

At its core, walking is a fundamental human movement that we often take for granted. Yet, by paying attention to the mechanics of each step, we can improve our posture, balance, and overall well-being. From the heel strike to the toe-off, each phase of the walking gait cycle offers an opportunity for refinement and efficiency.

Mindful walking, rooted in Buddhist traditions, encourages practitioners to bring awareness to each moment of movement. By focusing on the sensations of walking—the feeling of the ground beneath our feet, the rhythm of our breath, the sway of our body—we cultivate mindfulness and presence. This practice can be deeply grounding and transformative, offering a respite from the distractions of modern life.

Power walking, on the other hand, emphasizes speed and cardiovascular fitness. By walking at a brisk pace, engaging the arms, and maintaining proper form, enthusiasts can elevate their heart rate, burn calories, and strengthen muscles. Power walking is a popular choice for fitness enthusiasts of all ages, offering a low-impact alternative to running with similar benefits.

Walking meditation merges the principles of mindfulness with the act of walking. Practitioners often walk in a designated area, such as a garden or labyrinth, while maintaining awareness of their breath and bodily sensations. This moving meditation can be a powerful tool for stress reduction, self-reflection, and spiritual growth.

Regardless of the specific approach, walking steps invite us to reconnect with our bodies, our surroundings, and ourselves. Whether we're strolling through nature, navigating city streets, or pacing the halls of our home, each step holds the potential for exploration and discovery. So let's lace up our shoes, step outside, and embark on a journey of movement, mindfulness, and meaning.

Chapter 1

What Walking Means

Walking is a basic kind of human movement that is defined by a rhythmic step-by-step pattern. It is usually carried out standing up straight with one foot constantly on the ground. Through the coordinated use of muscles, joints, and sensory input, this kind of ambulation enables people to walk quickly and stably across short to intermediate distances. Walking is a major form of exercise, recreation, and transportation that promotes social connection, mental and physical health, and physical well-being.

The Art of Walking: Examining the Effortless yet Intense Act

In our fast-paced society, walking is often disregarded, yet it's a basic human activity that goes beyond simple transit. There are several physical and mental health advantages to walking, from fast urban commuting to relaxing walks in the outdoors. Together, we will investigate the art of walking and discover its basic but deep meaning in our lives.

2. An All-encompassing Language

Everyone can communicate via walking, regardless of background, age, or culture. It is a way of moving that is deeply rooted in our evolutionary history and that allows us to travel over terrain, interact with others, and discover our surroundings. Every step we take while walking, whether it's along peaceful woodland paths or meandering through busy city streets, enables us to soak in the rich tapestry of life.

3. Physical Health

Fundamentally, walking is a healthy workout that comes with several bodily advantages. Frequent walking improves cardiovascular health, builds muscular and bone strength, and enhances general fitness and energy. People of all ages and fitness levels may participate in walking since it is easy on the joints compared to more physically demanding hobbies. Even a little walk each day may have a big impact on our well-being, improving our mood, lowering our stress levels, and increasing our lifespan.

4. Intentional Movement

In the current world of endless stimulus and diversions, walking provides a unique chance for attentive movement. We might rediscover ourselves and our surroundings when we put down our devices and embrace the rhythm of walking. Every step we take grounds us in the present moment and turns it into a moment of presence. Amidst the craziness of everyday life, we may develop a feeling of calm, clarity, and inner balance by walking deliberately.

5. Investigation and Finding

Walking is a really enjoyable activity that allows for endless exploration and discovery. Walking provides many opportunities, whether we are exploring new ground or meandering through well-known districts. It asks us to pay attention to the little things that we would otherwise miss in our rushed lives, such as the brilliant colors of flowers in bloom, the soft rustling of leaves in the air, and the warm smiles of strangers.

6. Relationships and Community

Walking undoubtedly has the power to create a sense of community and connection by uniting individuals via similar experiences. Strolling offers an opportunity for social connection and companionship, ranging from casual walks with friends to formal walking clubs and neighborhood activities. We establish ties that cut across barriers and differences, have deep talks, and create new friendships as we stroll side by side.

In summary

Walking serves as a reminder to slow down, take deep breaths, and enjoy the little pleasures in life in a society that often values efficiency and speed. It is a celebration of our intrinsic capacity to move, explore, and interact with the world around us, and it is more than simply a way to travel from point A to point B. It is a deep statement of our humanity. Thus, put on your shoes, go outdoors, and welcome the art of walking. Who knows what treasures are ahead on your journey?

Chapter 2

Strolling methods and strolling at your speed are key to getting the most out of walking and making it enjoyable. The following methods and advice will help you walk efficiently and determine the ideal speed for you:

Walking Methods

1. Posture: Keep your shoulders back, head up, and abdomen engaged in an upright position. Steer clear of slouching or bending forward since this might put undue tension on your muscles and cause pain.

2. Walk: Step with ease and naturalness, letting your legs swing freely. Refrain from overstriding, since this may result in joint strain. With every stride, try to maintain a fluid, rhythmic gait.

3. Arm Swing: Maintain a comfortable, slightly angled posture while allowing your arms to swing freely at your sides. To keep your balance and momentum, make sure your arm and leg movements are in sync.

4. Foot Placement: Use your full foot to provide stability as you land on your heel and roll through to your toes with each stride. Stamping or slamming your feet should be avoided as this might put undue pressure and stress on your feet.

5. Breathing: As you walk, take deep, regular breaths from your nose and out through your mouth. To increase endurance and oxygenate your body, concentrate on deep belly breathing.

6. Cadence: For vigorous walking, aim for a steady cadence, or step rate, of 120 to 140 steps per minute. Try out several cadences to see which one is most effective and comfortable for you.

Choosing Your Speed:

1. Listen to Your Body: During your stroll, become aware of how your body feels. If you are experiencing pain, exhaustion, or shortness of breath, slow down or stop as required. It's important to pay attention to the cues your body gives you and modify your speed appropriately.

2. Start Slowly: If you've never walked before or are getting back into it after a hiatus, begin at a slower pace and progressively pick up more distance and speed over time. This lowers the chance of damage by enabling your body to gradually adjust and increase endurance.

3. Discover Your Comfort Zone: Try out various walking tempos to see what feels most sustainable and comfortable for you. While some individuals may enjoy a more leisurely walk, others would prefer a quick, athletic pace. Pick a speed that will enable you to continually enjoy the experience and keep it going.

4. Use a Pedometer or Fitness Tracker: To keep an eye on your steps, distance traveled, and pace, think about using a pedometer or fitness tracker. To enhance your walking performance, these gadgets may assist you in setting objectives, monitoring your development, and staying motivated.

5. Mindful Walking: When you walk, pay attention to your breathing patterns, the noises and images around you, and the sensations of your movement. This may support you in developing a calm and peaceful inner state of mind as well as helping you remain in the present.

6. Listen to Music or Podcasts: If you want to listen to music or podcasts while strolling, choose lively songs or interesting shows that will inspire you to keep going. You may also keep a steady pace by listening to music that has a constant speed.

You may make the most of your walking experience, improve your physical fitness, and take advantage of all the numerous advantages that walking has to offer by using these walking tactics and going at your speed. Whether you walk for physical activity, stress relief, or transit, always pay attention to your body, establish your rhythm, and take each step as it comes.

Chapter 3

Here are some pointers for optimizing your outdoor experiences:

1. Pick Your Destination: Do your homework and find a place that suits your tastes and interests. There is a place waiting to be discovered, whether you choose calm lakeside settings, expansive mountain views, or coastal beaches.

2. Make a Plan: Before leaving, familiarize yourself with park rules, trail conditions, and weather predictions. For any outdoor activities, make sure you have the right equipment, clothes, and supplies, such as water, food, sunscreen, and a map or GPS device.

3. Seize the Chance: Try new things or outdoor activities to get out of your comfort zone. Embracing adventure may result in thrilling

experiences and enduring memories, whether you're mountain biking, rock climbing, kayaking, or birding.

4. Unplug and Plug Back in: Give technology a rest and spend time entirely immersed in nature. Give up using social media and cell phones as distractions and concentrate on the sights, sounds, and feelings around you.

5. Put Leave No Trace Into Practice: Respect the environment and leave it in its original state by adhering to the Leave No Trace guidelines. To protect natural environments for future generations, remove any rubbish, leave as little trace as possible behind, and stick to established pathways.

6. Use Your Sensations: Enjoy the sensory experiences of being outside, such as the sound of birds singing, the warmth of the sun on your skin, and the aroma of wildflowers or pine trees. By using all of your senses, you may improve

your outdoor experience and strengthen your connection with the natural world.

7. Give It Some Thought: Make time to sit in silence and contemplate as you take in the beauty of your surroundings. These reflective moments may be calming and enlightening, whether they are spent sitting next to a peaceful stream, seeing the sunset, or staring up at a starry sky.

8. Talk About Your Experience: Bring loved ones, family, or friends along on your outdoor experiences. The happiness and companionship that come from being outside may be increased when you share the experience with others and make priceless memories that will last a lifetime.

9. Be Alert: When going on outdoor adventures, put safety first by keeping yourself informed, watching out for possible dangers, and taking preventative measures to lower the risk. Inform others of your goals and location, and if anything seems off, always follow your gut.

10. Construct a Conservation Legacy: Play a proactive part in conserving and safeguarding the environment so that future generations may enjoy it. Back conservation activities, lend a hand with neighborhood environmental projects and push for laws that protect the planet's priceless ecosystems.

Through a spirit of adventure, awareness, and stewardship, we may enter the great outdoors and uncover a world of inspiration, wonder, and discovery that feeds our body, mind, and soul. Put on your hiking boots, take your camera, and go on an outdoor experience that will make you appreciate the beauty of the environment and feel alive.

Chapter 4

Fitness and Well-Being Inside Four Walls: Embracing Indoor Walking

Although there's no denying the appeal of taking walks outside among the breathtaking scenery of nature, there are other advantages to walking inside, in our homes, or in other indoor areas. When the weather is bad, you're pressed for time, or you just prefer to walk inside, indoor walking is an easy and accessible option to maintain an active lifestyle and enhance general well-being. Let's investigate the benefits and pleasures of adopting indoor walking as a vital part of a healthy way of life.

Affordability and Availability

The ease of use and accessibility of indoor walking are among its greatest benefits. Walking inside eliminates worries about the weather, the time of day, and safety issues. Walking inside offers a dependable way to be active all year round, regardless of the weather—whether it's pouring, dark outdoors, or just too hot or cold outside. Furthermore, indoor walking is a simple habit to include in everyday schedules, whether it is as part of an organized fitness program, while watching television, or during work breaks.

Comfort and Safety

The regulated atmosphere that comes with walking inside puts comfort and safety first. Compared to outside walking on uneven ground, there is a lower chance of slips, trips, and falls on smooth, level surfaces and predictable terrain. For those with respiratory disorders, mobility issues, or sensitivity to outside factors, indoor walking is the best option since it reduces exposure to environmental risks like pollution, traffic, or allergies.

Adaptability and Originality

It's not always boring or monotonous to stroll inside, despite what the general public believes. Walking routines may be made far more creative and varied in indoor settings. Many indoor walking routines may be tailored to meet specific tastes and fitness objectives, ranging from walking laps around a large living room or hallway to climbing stairs, marching in place, or following along with indoor walking videos or fitness apps.

All Ages and Fitness Levels Can Access It

People of various ages, skills, and fitness levels may participate in indoor walking. Indoor walking may be tailored to accommodate a variety of goals and tastes, whether you're a seasoned athlete trying to maintain conditioning during bad weather or a newbie to exercise looking for a mild, low-impact sport. It offers a secure and efficient way for elderly people, those with limited mobility, or people recuperating from surgery or an accident to get

regular exercise and enjoy the health advantages
of walking.

Stress Reduction and Mental Health

Similar to walking outside, walking inside has
many advantages for mental health, such as
lowering stress, improving mood, and
stimulating the mind. Walking vigorously inside
may help reduce anxiety, stress, and restlessness
by generating endorphins, which are the body's
natural happy-making chemicals. In addition to
boosting mental clarity and emotional balance,
indoor walking offers a chance for mindfulness
and relaxation by enabling people to concentrate
on their breathing, movement, and
present-moment awareness.

Guides to Successful Indoor Walking

- Establish reasonable objectives and
progressively boost the time and intensity over
time.

- To keep your indoor walking regimen interesting and pleasurable, mix things up.
- Make an investment in cozy apparel and supportive shoes appropriate for working out inside.
-Employ audiobooks, podcasts, music, or virtual walking tours to boost your mood and level of motivation.
- For a comprehensive fitness program, think about adding stretching, strength training, or other complimentary workouts to your indoor walking routine.

Conclusion

Walking inside is a convenient and adaptable way to maintain an active, healthy, and joyful lifestyle even in situations when going outside isn't possible. People may enjoy the comforts and conveniences of indoor surroundings while walking and reap the many physical, mental, and emotional advantages of walking when they choose indoor walking as part of a balanced lifestyle. So put on your walking shoes, enter your house, and set off on a voyage of health and vigor within your four walls.